Guidance for Protecting Responders' Health During the First Week Following A Wide-Area Aerosol Anthrax Attack

Acronyms Used in this Document

ACIP	Advisory Committee on Immunization Practices
APR	Air Purifying Respirator
AVA	Anthrax Vaccine Adsorbed or BioThrax™
B. anthracis	*Bacillus anthracis*
CDC	Centers for Disease Control and Prevention
CFR	Code of Federal Regulations
CRI	Cities Readiness Initiative
DHS	US Department of Homeland Security
DOD	US Department of Defense
EUA	Emergency Use Authorization
FDA	Food and Drug Administration
HAZMAT	Hazardous Materials
HE	High Efficiency
HEPA	High Efficiency Particulate Air
HHS	US Department of Health and Human Services
IC	Incident Commander
IND	Investigational New Drug
MSA	Metropolitan Statistical Area
NIOSH	National Institute for Occupational Safety and Health
OSHA	Occupational Safety and Health Administration
PAPR	Powered Air Purifying Respirator
PEP	Post-exposure Prophylaxis
POD	Point of Dispensing
PPE	Personal Protective Equipment
SAR	Supplied Air Respirator
SCBA	Self-Contained Breathing Apparatus
SNS	Strategic National Stockpile
UC	Unified Command
US	United States
USPS	US Postal Service

I.   *Background*

A. *Purpose*

This guidance provides recommendations for protecting personnel responding to a wide-area anthrax attack from developing anthrax as a result of exposure to aerosolized *Bacillus anthracis* (*B. anthracis*) spores and for minimizing the amount of exposure in the first week of a response. This guidance has been requested by responders because the nature of their work may put them at higher risk of exposure when they are asked to enter contaminated areas and when their duties require them on an ongoing and repeated basis to interact with the environment in ways that may increase exposure. Protective measures include the same medical countermeasures (i.e., drugs, vaccine) that would be made available to the general population as well as personal protective equipment (PPE), and other possible work practices based on their job tasks. Guidance for a local population exposed to *B. anthracis* would come from their state and local governments; CDC has listed guidance for those governments at www.bt.cdc.gov/agent/anthrax/prep.

A federal interagency working group that included subject matter experts in biodefense, infectious diseases, and occupational health and safety developed this guidance regarding appropriate protective measures for responders in the immediate post-attack environment of a wide-area aerosol anthrax attack.

This guidance reflects the current understanding of the unique environment that would be expected during the first week of a wide-area anthrax release, and is expected to evolve with changes to our understanding regarding exposure risk, scientific developments, and availability of new environmental monitoring techniques. This guidance is intended to support ongoing planning and preparation efforts, as well as to lay the basis for plans to protect all individuals who may respond. This planning guidance will be refined as the evidence base for determining exposure risk and the efficacy of protective measures is strengthened.

Full implementation of the guidance presented in this document may be contingent upon the availability of sufficient supplies, such as vaccine for post-exposure prophylaxis. A federal interagency working group is currently developing a post-exposure vaccine prioritization policy for both exposure risk and vaccine availability. This guidance document, therefore, will be refined and adjusted to reflect prioritization recommendations upon completion of that policy.

This guidance is not meant to supplant other existing guidance or the judgment of incident commanders or responders who are on the scene of an actual incident and who may have access to specific data that can enable more informed decision-making.

B. *Defining Responders*

This guidance defines "responders" as a diverse set of individuals who are critical to mitigating the potential catastrophic effects of a wide-area aerosol anthrax attack. This broad definition includes professional and traditional first responders (e.g., emergency medical services practitioners, firefighters, law enforcement, and HAZMAT personnel); the emergency management community; public health and medical professionals; skilled support personnel; and emergency service and critical infrastructure personnel. Responders may be from government, volunteer, or private sector organizations.

C. Wide-Area Aerosol Anthrax Attack Scenario

This guidance was developed to address a particular scenario: the first week following a wide-area aerosol anthrax attack in a large U.S. city. Such an attack employing *B. anthracis* spores would present different challenges than would a smaller scale or indoor anthrax attack or an attack involving other biological agents. Specifically, this guidance applies to a scenario in which a quantity of *B. anthracis* spores is disseminated as a small-particle aerosol generated by a spraying device. The spores could be released from a single point or along a dissemination line from either a ground-based (e.g., truck-mounted sprayer) or an airborne (e.g., crop duster) delivery vehicle. The affected area could encompass hundreds of square miles and could potentially expose hundreds of thousands of people to spores, which, once inhaled, could cause extensive illness and death in the affected population. The assumptions used to address underlying uncertainties associated with this scenario are listed in Appendix 1.

D. The Response

To frame the guidance for protecting responders' health during the first week following a wide-area aerosol anthrax attack, it is important to review and understand current plans and recommendations for mitigating the health effects in the general population suspected of exposure. The successful execution of a wide-area aerosol anthrax attack in a major metropolitan area could have disastrous effects. The risk of fatality associated with inhalation anthrax can be extremely high, particularly among those who do not initiate a post-exposure prophylaxis (PEP) regimen before symptoms develop; therefore, a primary response goal is to ensure rapid distribution of PEP to the impacted population.

Current recommendations for PEP for the general population can be found at www.cdc.gov/mmwr/preview/mmwrhtml/rr5906a1.htm. They include the timely administration of a minimum 60-day course of oral antimicrobial drugs (e.g., doxycycline or ciprofloxacin) following potential or imminent exposure to *B. anthracis* spores in combination with three doses of anthrax vaccine adsorbed (AVA, BioThrax™), given subcutaneously at 0, 2, and 4 weeks for those not previously vaccinated.

Anthrax vaccine is presently licensed by the Food and Drug Administration (FDA) for anthrax pre-exposure prophylaxis for persons at high risk of anthrax exposure. Anthrax vaccine is routinely given to researchers, certain laboratory personnel, some military personnel, and people who handle animals or animal products such as some veterinarians. The regimen for pre-exposure prophylaxis is a five-dose series followed by annual boosters.

Although anthrax vaccine is not licensed for post-exposure use, its use as a component of PEP could be authorized by the FDA under an Emergency Use Authorization (EUA) during an emergency declared by the Secretary of HHS justifying such authorization for those 18 years of age and older. For those under 18 years of age, vaccine could be provided under an Investigational New Drug (IND) protocol. Human and animal data suggest that the oral antimicrobial component of PEP provides the best protection when started as early as possible after exposure to spores and before the onset of clinical symptoms. This guidance uses a 48-hour timeline between exposure and the potential onset of symptoms. Meeting this timeline increases the ability to save lives, maintain social order, avoid significant economic loss, ensure continuity of government, and preserve the public's confidence in the government's ability to respond to an attack.

There are significant logistical challenges to ensuring an effective response in the wake of a wide-area anthrax attack. Because oral antimicrobial drugs are most effective for anthrax prophylaxis when administered prior to the onset of symptoms, and because a wide-area aerosol release of *B. anthracis* spores may go undetected for hours or even days, the time available to distribute and dispense these oral antimicrobial drugs is short. Additionally, in the early days of the incident, determining who was or was not exposed to anthrax spores will be difficult. Environmental monitoring and early detection capabilities for certain biological agents are already fielded in our nation's largest cities. However, current technologies do not provide instantaneous results; they require time for both sampling and analysis. If an attack were to occur beyond the range of one of these systems, its detection would likely depend on clinical diagnosis after people begin to seek medical treatment for symptoms. In such cases, the time remaining to effectively protect the affected population is even more limited. It may be necessary, therefore, to distribute PEP to the entire population in the area with the understanding that, as characterization data are gathered, PEP recommendations may be modified.

The Centers for Disease Control and Prevention's (CDC) Strategic National Stockpile (SNS) has quantities of medicine and medical supplies to provide for the emergency health security of the United States. The SNS may be deployed as required by the Secretary of the Department of Homeland Security (DHS) to respond to an actual or potential emergency, or at the discretion of the Secretary of HHS to respond to an actual or potential public health emergency or other situation in which the deployment is necessary to protect the public health or safety. When authorities agree that the SNS is needed, medical countermeasures can be delivered to any state in the United States (US) within hours. CDC's Cities Readiness Initiative (CRI) is a federally funded program designed to enhance preparedness in the nation's largest cities and Metropolitan Statistical Areas (MSA) where more than half of the US population resides. Through CRI, state and large metropolitan public health departments have developed plans to respond to a large-scale anthrax event by dispensing antimicrobial drugs to the entire population of an identified MSA within 48 hours.

Each state has plans to receive and distribute antimicrobial drugs for PEP to local communities as quickly as possible. Most jurisdictional plans for dispensing oral antimicrobial drugs involve the establishment of community Points of Dispensing

(PODs), although several jurisdictions are in the active planning stages to employ the postal model for rapid distribution of PEP as a complement to PODs. On notification, PODs or US Postal Service assets would be established to receive antimicrobial drugs and dispense them to the potentially exposed population.

Employer organizations from which responders originate may consider actions to cache oral antimicrobial drugs before an incident for dispensing to responders immediately post-event. Employers may refer to the FDA's emergency use authorization (EUA) which allows for the pre-event stockpiling of doxycycline. (See www.fda.gov/EmergencyPreparedness/Counterterrorism/ucm269226.htm) The goals of pre-event placement of oral antimicrobial drugs are to: 1) ensure continuation of mission-essential functions by avoiding the time lag of acquiring, distributing, and dispensing oral antimicrobial drugs, and 2) lessen the workload of dispensing oral antimicrobial drugs to the general public post-event. Dispensing of cached oral antimicrobial drugs may occur under either a medical or a non-medical dispensing model. A medical model involves pre-screening of potential recipients for appropriate oral antimicrobial drug use, dosing, contraindications, and other criteria. In a non-medical dispensing model, limited health and demographic data are gathered prior to dispensing PEP; such models are in place in many communities to serve the general population.

Employers and organizations from which responders originate need to make available PPE and educate responders about appropriate PPE consistent with National Institute for Occupational Safety and Health (NIOSH) and Occupational Safety and Health Administration (OSHA) regulations and guidance based on activities expected to be performed. See additional resources in Appendix 2.

II.   *Protecting Responders*

To protect their health immediately following a wide-area aerosol anthrax attack, all possible measures need to be taken to minimize responders' exposure to *B. anthracis* spores. For most common hazards and usual exposure scenarios, this would be accomplished using primary interventions such as engineering controls (e.g., safe havens, isolation, and ventilation), work practice modifications, limiting access to and duration in the affected area, and proper use and selection of appropriate PPE. If the source of the hazard and extent of the contamination can be predicted or directly measured, then these data can form the basis for assessing responder risk and selecting protective measures appropriate for each contaminated area and situation.

In the case of a wide-area release of aerosolized *B. anthracis*, it will likely be necessary to dispatch responders before it is possible to delineate specific areas contaminated with *B. anthracis* spores. Such a scenario is premised on an assumed delay (i.e., 12-36 hours or longer) between the time of an attack and recognition that an attack has occurred; therefore, primary controls for response personnel residing within the contaminated area will almost certainly not be implemented in time to prevent initial spore inhalation among some responders. For this scenario, there are adjunct measures to minimize the level of additional exposure responders receive, thereby reducing any added risk for infection. Incident commanders (IC) need to recognize the potential inherent risk of exposure to those not exposed during the original attack, and must ensure that appropriate protective measures are initiated as part of coordinating response actions.

The ability to determine exposure risk will be limited, and exposure will likely not be uniform for responders, even among those residing inside the affected area. Some local responders may not have been exposed during the attack (e.g., if they live upwind of the aerosol release, were indoors in a controlled environment at the time of attack, were out of town on the day of attack, or live in an unaffected area). This guidance outlines PEP, PPE, and other protective measures that are needed to both reduce the probability of exposure and to decrease the risk to those who have been exposed.

Employers and organizations from which responders originate need to ensure that emergency response plans address emergency medical treatment and first aid for responders. In addition, responders need to be provided access to medical examinations and consultations if they become injured, develop signs or symptoms of exposure to hazardous substances, or experience adverse events associated with prophylaxis, per requirements set forth in 29 CFR 1910.120(f). Medical examinations and consultations need to be provided as soon as possible following the incident and at additional times if a physician determines it is necessary.

Prior to potential exposure, all personnel who will respond to a wide-area aerosol anthrax attack need to be trained on the hazards of *B. anthracis* exposure and how to reduce these hazards: specifically, they need to be trained on the routes of transmission, the signs and symptoms of anthrax, the morbidity and mortality associated with various types of anthrax, any medical conditions which would place responders at increased risk for developing anthrax, and protective measures to reduce exposure to *B. anthracis* spores. Training on protective measures to reduce exposure shall include information on appropriate engineering controls, work practices, housekeeping, and proper use and selection of appropriate PPE and proper decontamination techniques of both PPE and personnel.

A. Oral Antimicrobial Drug Component of Post-Exposure Prophylaxis (PEP)

After being inhaled into the lungs, *B. anthracis* spores are transported to regional lymph nodes where they can germinate into toxin-producing bacteria. The bacteria and toxins cause systemic anthrax. Spores may germinate in one or a few days, but some spores can remain dormant for weeks or months before germinating. Animal models of spore germination for inhalation anthrax and clearance kinetics suggest that complete clearance may take 60 days or longer.

To prevent or arrest development of symptoms of anthrax, oral antimicrobial drugs will be made available as soon as possible for all individuals in the population who could have been subjected to the initial aerosol exposure. Response workers will be given antimicrobial drugs, including workers exposed during the initial incident as well as those workers who could potentially be exposed to *B. anthracis* as a function of their work duties. Unvaccinated response workers must begin oral PEP before exposure if they will be working in an environment where spore release is suspected to have occurred; if that is not possible, they should begin as soon as possible after their first suspected exposure.

The oral antimicrobial component of PEP is the foundation of protection. The antimicrobial drugs ciprofloxacin and doxycycline are equally effective against naturally occurring strains of *B. anthracis* and are currently the two first-line drugs of choice for PEP. Either ciprofloxacin (500 milligrams twice a day) or doxycycline (100 milligrams twice a day) is recommended for all responders who are not fully vaccinated (i.e., completed the five-dose vaccine series or who have not maintained annual boosters). For maximum potential protection, these antimicrobial drugs should be initiated as soon as possible after the potential exposure. In the absence of vaccination, antimicrobial drugs should be continued for 60 days after the last possible exposure. For recommendations for antimicrobial PEP in the setting of post-exposure vaccination, see the following section on the anthrax vaccine component of PEP.

The combination of pre-event vaccine and appropriate PPE effectively protects fully vaccinated persons who work in occupations that might result in repeated exposure to aerosolized *B. anthracis* spores. Antimicrobial PEP is not needed for fully vaccinated workers who wear appropriate PPE while working in environments contaminated with *B. anthracis* spores unless the PPE is disrupted. The CDC's Advisory Committee on Immunization Practices (ACIP) (CDC, 2010) suggests that the threshold for assuming PPE has been compromised should be extremely low. Fully vaccinated workers who prefer additional protection may consider antimicrobial PEP under the direction of their occupational health program. A 30-day course of antimicrobial PEP is recommended for partially vaccinated workers, fully vaccinated workers who do not wear PPE, and fully vaccinated workers who's PPE has been disrupted; these workers should continue with their licensed vaccination regimen. (CDC, 2010)

B.   *Anthrax Vaccine Component of PEP*

According to the recommendations of the ACIP, all personnel who have been potentially exposed and have not been previously fully vaccinated should be considered for post-exposure vaccination as soon as it is made available, using a three-dose regimen administered subcutaneously, in addition to the recommended oral antimicrobial PEP regimen described above. The first vaccine dose should be administered as soon as possible post-exposure; the second and third doses should be administered two and four weeks after the first dose is administered. Coordination for making available and receiving post-exposure vaccination should be made through departments of health.

Anthrax vaccine is not immediately effective. Therefore, in a post-exposure setting, a combination of an oral antimicrobial drug and anthrax vaccination (i.e., PEP) offers the best potential protection for those exposed to an aerosol *B. anthracis* release. When vaccine is used along with oral antimicrobial drugs for PEP, CDC recommends that oral antimicrobial drugs be taken until the vaccine is expected to be protective (i.e., 14 days after the third vaccine dose).

Depending on the size of the populations exposed and the availability of vaccine, vaccine may need to be prioritized. A prioritization policy for vaccine for PEP for the general population and responders, for use when applicable, is currently under development by a federal interagency group. Once published, incident commanders and decision-makers should familiarize themselves with the policy.

C. Personal Protective Equipment (PPE)

All employers and organizations sponsoring responders have an obligation to lessen the risk of illness and death among responders by providing appropriate PPE and associated training to reduce hazard exposure. In addition to taking oral antimicrobial PEP, responders need to adhere to applicable requirements, and if such requirements do not exist, to existing recommendations related to the use of PPE when working in a contaminated environment. PPE includes appropriate respiratory protection, protective garments, and nitrile or vinyl gloves.

Because data are lacking regarding oral antimicrobial efficacy in the setting of repeated exposure to *B. anthracis* spores and the impact of total spore burden, PPE needs to be used to minimize the continued inhalational burden of *B. anthracis* spores. Procedures for the use of PPE are based on an understanding of potential environmental contamination, risk of exposure, exposure pathway, and anticipated level of exposure. In the absence of information specific to contamination levels and potential for re-aerosolization, it is prudent to believe that some activities conducted in contaminated areas may increase the probable level of exposure. Therefore, PPE is needed initially to reduce responder exposures until the results of risk assessments are available. OSHA may be requested to assist in post-event assessments of health and safety hazards of the incident environment. Once hazards have been assessed, OSHA can expeditiously convene experts to provide further guidance on protective measures for various post-event activities.

A full facepiece air purifying respirator (APR) with P100 or N100 filters or a full facepiece powered air purifying respirator (PAPR) with high efficiency (HE) filters offers protection against inhalation exposure to *B. anthracis* spores. This equipment may be needed for certain high-risk activities, including environmental sampling and remediation activities. Higher levels of protection, such as chemical, biological, radiological, and nuclear (CBRN) rated self-contained breathing apparatus (SCBA), are only needed when there may be an ongoing release using an aerosol-generating device or when the agent is unknown.

Depending on the activities being performed by the responder, some level of protection from dermal exposure may be warranted. When exposure is expected, it is recommended that disposable hooded coveralls, gloves, and foot coverings be used. In some settings, however, changing the outer layer of clothing may be sufficient.

When mandated by IC as part of a Unified Command (UC) or other incident management system, PPE including respiratory protection needs to be employed in accordance with OSHA standards and regulations found in 29 CFR Part 1910 Subpart I (1910.132—1910.138) or the equivalent construction standards (29 CFR Part 1926). These standards require training on the proper selection, use, removal, and disposal of PPE; a medical evaluation and fit-testing must be conducted prior to use of any respiratory protection and annually thereafter.

D. Personal Decontamination and Hygiene

The extent of personal contamination for those working in an area suspected of being contaminated will not be known. During the activities with the highest risk of exposure, the outermost surfaces of protective clothing and gear will probably be contaminated with spores. Appropriate decontamination procedures are necessary to prevent these spores from being disseminated to less contaminated zones or areas by responder movement. (See 29 CFR 1910.120(k) for detailed guidance.) Appropriate decontamination can also reduce the potential hazard to household members associated with bringing contaminated items into a responder's home.

IC or public health authorities should determine locations, facilities, and specific decontamination procedures for this highest risk group. At the end of a shift or more often if needed, responders should undergo appropriate decontamination procedures, correctly remove and dispose of protective clothing, shoe coverings, and undergarments. Responders should then shower with soap and water and wash their hair.

In areas where the IC or UC has not prescribed the use of PPE, rigorous decontamination procedures are not required. However, use of normal hygiene procedures including hand washing and showering would provide some benefit in the event that surface contamination was present. Additional information regarding decontamination can be found in Appendix 2 (Resources 7, 8, 10, 11, and 12).

E. Administrative and Engineering Controls

Administrative and engineering controls can be effective when there is knowledge of the locations and activities that could possibly constitute an increased hazard. Administrative controls are frequently used where hazards are not particularly well-controlled and may include limiting tours of duty to reduce the duration a responder is exposed and limiting the number of responders working in the contaminated area. Administrative controls also could include deploying responders who have been vaccinated previously and are presumably at lower risk of developing illness. Another administrative control would be to discourage activities that may re-suspend settled spores and generate aerosols. Dust control measures, such as dust suppression with a water mist, may also help reduce re-aerosolization.

Engineering controls may include removing a hazard or placing a barrier between the worker and the hazard. Well-designed engineering controls can be highly effective in protecting workers. Examples may include placing impermeable physical barriers or encapsulants between responders and contaminated items. Other controls to reduce exposure could include using high efficiency particulate air (HEPA) vacuums in contaminated areas or using local exhaust ventilation, although such strategies may be limited or less practical in a wide-area release.

NIOSH published a document, *Guidance for Filtration and Air-Cleaning Systems to Protect Building Environments from Airborne Chemical, Biological, or Radiological Attacks*. This document describes preventive measures that building owners and managers can implement to protect building air environments from a terrorist release of chemical, biological, or radiological contaminants.

F. Pre-Event Vaccination

In July 2009, the CDC's Advisory Committee on Immunization Practices (ACIP) stated that by priming the immune system before exposure to *B. anthracis* spores, pre-event and pre-exposure vaccination might provide more protection than antimicrobial drugs alone to persons at risk for occupational exposure to *B. anthracis*. The ACIP stated that emergency and other responders are not recommended to receive routine pre-event vaccination because of the lack of a calculable risk assessment. However, if responder organizations undertake response activities that can lead to exposure to aerosolized *B. anthracis* spores and offer their workers pre-event vaccination on a voluntary basis in the context of an occupational health program, they should do so based on a calculated risk assessment. In the absence of such an assessment, vaccination may be considered based on an estimated or presumed risk-benefit assessment. Guidance is presently being developed for considering pre-event anthrax vaccination for first responders who would be engaged in response activities to an anthrax event.

Adverse events associated with vaccination may be reported to the Vaccine Adverse Event Reporting system which may be found at www.vaers.hhs.gov.

III. Exposure Risk Categories

Risk assessment is a structured approach to assessing vulnerability and defining appropriate protective measures based on anticipated hazards. This guidance is based on such a risk-based approach to preparedness, which takes into consideration factors such as the timing, duration, and potential level of exposure; the specific activities to be undertaken; and the anthrax vaccination status of the responder. Responder activities can be categorized based on the likelihood of exposure to *B. anthracis* spores. An individual's risk of illness should be characterized based on the highest risk of exposure associated with the activities anticipated on the part of that responder. Given the inherent uncertainties in assigning exposure risk, a balanced and precautionary approach is recommended.

In the absence of a reliable mechanism to immediately measure exposure over space and time, estimates of exposure rely on the assumptions that concentrations of spores are likely to be highest at the point or along the line of first release and diminish at some rate at points away or downwind from the release site. It is assumed that the rate of re-aerosolization will decrease by several orders of magnitude as time after initial particle deposition increases. There is convincing scientific evidence (Weis CP et al., 2002) to state that *Bacillus* spores, like any other small particle, can be re-aerosolized off surfaces due to natural forces and human activity. Additionally, in the first days following a release, some hazard associated with mechanically induced resuspension (e.g., vehicle traffic) may also be a concern. Particularly in the first few days of the response, it cannot be ruled out that some level of exposure risk may increase with travel frequency and duration into one or multiple potentially contaminated areas. There is some evidence (Los Alamos National Laboratories, 2011) that suggests relatively significant resuspension of spores as a result of mechanical disturbance; however, the resuspension seems to diminish over a relatively short time period.

Scientific research is being conducted to better define these variables. Even with limited initial knowledge of the extent of contamination, developing an activity-based approach to classifying potential risk among responders is possible. For instance, the highest-risk activities that responders engage in are likely to be: environmental or forensics sampling, decontamination activities, and other duties occurring within suspected contaminated areas. Those responders performing these activities would comprise the group that has the highest risk.

As more data become available, IC or other decision-makers may be able to refine their guidance, making site-based and activity-based decisions regarding appropriate protective measures to be employed. These decisions should be based on factors related to the specific incident, consultation with public health and occupational safety and health professionals, and additional knowledge obtained over the course of the response. Incident commanders, other incident leaders, employers, and public health authorities should consider additional information (e.g., sampling data and analyses and witnessed release locations) as it becomes available when recommending or selecting specific protective measures for responders following an attack.

It is prudent to assume that the responder population exposed or potentially exposed to the primary aerosol release will be at risk of illness during the first week after the attack. The primary exposure is believed to lead to a higher dose of *B. anthracis* spores than does secondary exposure. All personnel, regardless of whether their exposure is felt to be primary or secondary, should receive PEP medical countermeasures. Personnel should follow public health recommendations for PEP, consistent with the responder's vaccination status. For the majority of responders, these recommendations include oral antimicrobial drugs and vaccine, as described above.

A. Category 1 Activities – Highest Risk of Exposure During Responder Activities

Responders performing Category 1, or highest risk, activities will likely encounter high potential for exposure to spores, increasing the risk for inhalation or cutaneous anthrax. The highest potential exposure levels should be assumed for those performing activities in areas that are identified as the point of initial release and those activities that may involve prolonged contact with potentially contaminated surfaces, contaminant sampling, environmental remediation, forensic investigations, and spore re-aerosolization tasks. Personnel who perform these tasks may include HAZMAT teams, law enforcement and contractors performing remediation services.

B. Category 2 Activities – Variable/Unknown Risk of Exposure, but not Highest Potential Exposure Levels During Responder Activities

Following the initial primary aerosol release, exposures to secondary aerosols may occur through re-aerosolization of settled spores from surfaces. The extent of this secondary aerosol exposure will be unpredictable, difficult to quantify, and will vary depending on proximity and temporal relationship to the original release site, characteristics and quantity of the original source material, meteorological conditions, types of surfaces contaminated, and the activities being conducted. There is evidence to suggest that secondary exposures may have lower infectious dose exposures than do primary exposures.

Variable and unknown exposure levels that are not associated with high-exposure activities should be assumed for responders performing Category 2, or variable/unknown risk , activities in close proximity to, but not in, areas identified as contaminated by the initial release and for responders working in areas contaminated through secondary contamination confirmed by sampling. Exposure to re-aerosolized spores and contaminated surfaces is possible for responders performing Category 2 activities who are not expected to perform aerosol-generating work activities. Responders performing Category 2 activities may include, but are not limited to, law enforcement personnel; emergency medical services; firefighters; postal delivery staff and security escorts; public health staff; essential staff maintaining critical infrastructure operations; hospital staff; and mission-critical local, state, tribal, territorial, and federal personnel.

Responders who were originally exposed to the primary aerosol (e.g., during a Category 1 activity or before beginning the response) should be prioritized for PEP ahead of responders not exposed to the primary release and prior to conducting any further response activities. As guidance is developed and published for considering pre-event anthrax vaccination for certain responders, incident commanders should first consider deploying those responders who have been pre-vaccinated and are current in their vaccination schedule before employing unvaccinated responders. Recordkeeping of responders' activities and locations is encouraged so that, as information about the incident unfolds, the extent of total potential exposure among responders can be estimated.

When a risk assessment has been conducted by the employer, responders may use alternate PPE. In certain specialized situations after consideration of factors described below, half-mask elastomeric respirators with a filter cartridge (e.g., N95 or P100) or filtering facepiece respirators in conjunction with reduced levels of dermal protection may be considered, but it should be recognized that this level of PPE may not provide sufficient exposure reduction for many situations. Several parameters should be assessed when making a decision to downgrade the ensemble. These include knowledge of the source and extent of contamination, the level of uncertainty in the risk assessment, specific activities to be conducted, contingency or backup plans, length of time in the contaminated area, and provision for immunization and PEP. A decision of this nature should be carefully evaluated and made by industrial hygiene, safety, and medical personnel in conjunction with the incident commander and other appropriate public health authorities.

Table 1 summarizes the guidance on protective measures for responders performing Category 1 and 2 activities.

Table 1.

Protecting Responders' Health Based on Risk Category of Activities

Protective Measure	Guidance for Responders Performing Category 1 Activities	Guidance for Responders Performing Category 2 Activities
Post-Exposure Prophylaxis Antimicrobial Drugs	• Recommended for all responders who have not been fully vaccinated previously and for those who have been fully vaccinated but whose PPE has been disrupted • Begin regimen as soon as possible before or after initial exposure	
Post-Exposure Vaccination	• Yes, at the recommendation of public health officials and according to vaccine availability	
Personal Protective Equipment	• Level C protective ensemble with a full facepiece air purifying respirator (APR) with P100 or N100 filters *OR* Level C protective ensemble with a full facepiece powered air purifying respirator (PAPR) equipped with high efficiency (HE) filters • Disposable hooded coveralls and shoe coverings • Nitrile or vinyl gloves	• PPE, including respiratory protection and protective clothing, may be required *Note: Appropriate risk assessments will be performed at the time of the event to select the necessary PPE, informed by responder activities, proximity to the release and/or other confirmed contaminated areas, and specific event information available at the time. The use of PPE at the time of the event should be precautionary, with higher levels of PPE used until the response data indicate otherwise. When sufficient data and information are available, the assessment should be repeated with a focus on activities.* *Examples of PPE appropriate for Category 2 activities include filtering facepiece respirators and gloves for responders contacting potentially contaminated surfaces or items.*
Personal Decontamination / Hygiene	• After appropriate decontamination procedures, correctly remove and dispose of protective clothing • Dispose of undergarments worn under protective clothing • Shower with soap and water and wash hair • Depending on the type of respirator worn, decontaminate or dispose of respiratory protection *Note: Elastomeric respirators are amenable to decontamination. See EPA information in Appendix 2.*	

Appendix 1.   Scenario, Impact, and Response Assumptions

This guidance is intended to facilitate planning for one particular scenario, a wide-area aerosol anthrax attack. This scenario is based on a number of assumptions about the nature of the attack and the resulting environmental contamination. These parameters may vary in a real event, particularly as the event evolves and further characterization of the extent of the attack and other specific information is gained. Furthermore, the guidance may change based on changes in our understanding of the behavior of the contaminant, availability of monitoring and analytic technologies, and our understanding of the availability and efficacy of the protective measures recommended. The most important of the assumptions associated with this guidance are listed below:

Assumptions regarding attack scenario: (NOTE: assumptions are made for planning purposes and might not hold in a specific future incident)

- The attack involves only a single threat agent, *B. anthracis.*
- This guidance applies to a scenario in which a quantity of *B. anthracis* spores in a liquid or dried preparation is disseminated as a small-particle aerosol generated by a spraying device.
- The release is outdoors, contaminating a wide area, using *B. anthracis.*
- Wide-area environmental contamination is possible; this contamination will be spotty and not accurately predicted by models.
- The strain of *B. anthracis* used in the attack has not been modified or engineered to express resistance to oral antimicrobial drugs. To date, naturally occurring strains of *B. anthracis* are susceptible to ciprofloxacin and doxycycline.
- The aerosol attack is covert; initial notification will occur after environmental sensors, disease manifestation, or credible forensic intelligence provide evidence of or detect the presence of *B. anthracis* spores.

Assumptions regarding ability to characterize environmental distribution:

- BioWatch or other detection systems may not recognize the attack.
- Environmental monitoring and forensic efforts will be unable to provide timely information regarding the release, source strength, and scope/area of risk.
- Modeling is unable to accurately predict the specific area of risk from primary aerosol exposure but will be of value to incident commanders attempting to characterize the scope of the attack.
- Uncertainty about the extent of contamination and associated risk for the first week (or more) exists owing to the complexity of the problem and current (and foreseeable) capacity for sampling and testing.
- Travel within the geographical area could increase the likelihood of additional aerosol exposure by inadvertent entry into areas of high contamination or susceptibility of spore re-aerosolization.
- People transiting into and out of the potentially affected area will complicate risk assessment and potentially increase the spread of contamination.

- Demand for oral antimicrobial drugs and vaccine will likely extend beyond the geographic boundaries of the affected area. Environmental hazard mapping will be undertaken immediately, but may not be able to fully assess the potential contaminated area.
- Changes in environmental conditions, such as wind and rain, may complicate risk assessment and the potential spread of contamination.

Assumptions regarding impact to the population suspected to be exposed:

- By the time an attack has been recognized, regardless of detection mechanism, people may have been traveling in and out of affected areas for 36 hours or more.
- Everyone within the suspected area of contamination is considered to be at some level of risk of exposure (either primary or secondary) for the entire duration of their presence in the area, although the specific risk is not predictable.
- A large number of people in a broad geographical area will inhale *B. anthracis* spores but it will not be possible to determine specifically which people are exposed and will develop an infection; therefore, all people suspected of exposure will require a post-exposure regimen of 60 days of appropriate oral antimicrobial PEP, and should be considered for a three-dose regimen of anthrax vaccine.

Assumptions regarding response:

- The emergency use of certain medical countermeasures will be authorized under EUAs following specific steps by the Secretaries of HHS, DHS, or Department of Defense (DOD) to make a specific emergency determination; by the HHS Secretary to make a declaration justifying the emergency use of the product; and by the FDA to issue each EUA. (An EUA for oral formulations of doxycycline products for PEP of inhalation anthrax was issued by FDA in July 2011, to facilitate anthrax preparedness and response efforts.)
- Modalities (e.g., public health PODs, retail PODS, employer PODs) will be activated following an attack to dispense oral antimicrobial drugs to the at-risk population as quickly as possible.
- The immediate dispensing of oral antimicrobial drugs to the at-risk population may also rely on a venue-specific Postal Plan that involves postal carrier volunteers with law enforcement escorts delivering oral antimicrobial drugs or other "push" options under local jurisdictional consideration.
- Many responders originate from inside the at-risk geographic area, and therefore will have been at risk of exposure from the primary aerosol.
- All transportation in and proximal to the aerosol release will be affected.
- Responders who originate from outside the affected geographic area will be moving from a status of essentially no likely exposure into an area that places them at increased risk for exposure to *B. anthracis* spores through secondary aerosolization.
- In addition to traditional "first responders," a number of other responders will be critical during the first week following an anthrax attack, including essential employees across critical infrastructure sectors who must provide uninterrupted

services immediately following an attack (e.g., hospital and nursing home staff, public health staff and volunteers, prison guards, airport security, border guards, and those staffing telecommunications, electrical power, and water facilities).

- In addition to concerns related to actual exposure of the population and responders, there could be significant concern within both groups about possible and undetected exposure. Effectively managing this concern may require behavioral health intervention in addition to medical triage and intervention.

Appendix 2. Sources of Additional Information

Note: All links were current as of August 2012.

1. ***Anthrax***
   Centers for Disease Control and Prevention, 2011
   www.bt.cdc.gov/agent/anthrax

2. ***Anthrax eTool: Protecting the Worksite against Terrorism***
   Occupational Safety and Health Administration, 2011
   www.osha.gov/SLTC/etools/anthrax/ppe.html

3. ***Anthrax Spore Decontamination Using Bleach (Sodium Hypochlorite)***
   Environmental Protection Agency, 2007
   www.epa.gov/pesticides/factsheets/chemicals/bleachfactsheet.htm

4. ***Guidance for Filtration and Air-Cleaning Systems to Protect Building Environments from Airborne Chemical, Biological, or Radiological Attacks***
   National Institute for Occupational Safety and Health, 2003
   www.cdc.gov/niosh/docs/2003-136

5. ***Guidance on Emergency Responder Personal Protective Equipment (PPE) for Response to CBRN Terrorism Incidents***
   National Institute for Occupational Safety and Health, 2008
   www.cdc.gov/niosh/programs/ppt/pdfs/PPE_Interim_Guidance_6-10-08.pdf

6. ***Interim Questions and Answers: Emergency Use Authorization for Oral Formulations of Doxycycline for Post-Exposure Prophylaxis of Inhalational Anthrax***
   Food and Drug Administration, 2012
   www.fda.gov/EmergencyPreparedness/Counterterrorism/ucm269226.htm

7. ***NFPA 472: Standard for Competence of Responders to Hazardous Materials/Weapons of Mass Destruction Incidents***
   National Fire Protection Association, 2008
   www.nfpa.org/aboutthecodes/AboutTheCodes.asp?DocNum=472&cookie%5Ftest=1

8. ***Occupational Health Guidelines for Remediation Workers at* Bacillus anthracis-*Contaminated Sites—United States, 2001–2002***
   Centers for Disease Control and Prevention, 2002
   www.cdc.gov/mmwr/preview/mmwrhtml/mm5135a3.htm

9. *Planning Guidance for Recovery Following Biological Incidents (DRAFT), Appendix 5*
    Environmental Protection Agency, Department of Homeland Security, 2011
    www.regulations.gov/contentStreamer?objectId=0900006480a03c20&disposition=attachment&contentType=pdf

10. *Protecting Emergency Responders*
    National Institute for Occupational Safety and Health and RAND Corp., 2002
    www.rand.org/publications/CF/CF176

11. *Protecting Investigators Performing Environmental Sampling for* **Bacillus anthracis***: Personal Protective Equipment*
    Centers for Disease Control and Prevention, 2001
    http://www.bt.cdc.gov/agent/anthrax/environment/investigatorppe.asp

12. *Recommendations for the Selection and Use of Respirators and Protective Clothing for Protection against Biological Agents*
    National Institute for Occupational Safety and Health, 2009
    www.cdc.gov/niosh/docs/2009-132

13. *Responding to Detection of Aerosolized* **Bacillus anthracis** *by Autonomous Detection Systems in the Workplace*
    Centers for Disease Control and Prevention, 2004
    www.cdc.gov/mmwr/preview/mmwrhtml/rr5307a1.htm

14. *Safety and Health Topics: Anthrax*
    Occupational Safety and Health Administration, 2011
    www.osha.gov/SLTC/bioterrorism/anthrax/index.html

15. *Use of Anthrax Vaccine in the United States; Recommendations of the Advisory Committee on Immunizations Practices (ACIP), 2009*
    Centers for Disease Control and Prevention, 2010
    www.cdc.gov/mmwr/pdf/rr/rr5906.pdf

Appendix 3.   References Cited in the Text

Centers for Disease Control and Prevention. Use of Anthrax Vaccine in the United States: Recommendations of the Advisory Committee on Immunization Practices (ACIP), 2009. MMWR 2010;59(No. RR-6).

Los Alamos National Laboratories. (2011). *Bacillus anthracis* outdoor secondary aerosolization (reaerosolization): annotated bibliography. Washington, DC. Government Printing Office.

Weis CP, Intrepido AJ, Miller AK, et al. Secondary aerosolization of viable *Bacillus anthracis* spores in a contaminated US Senate office. JAMA. 2002;288(22):2853-2858.

Page Intentionally Left Blank

www.ingramcontent.com/pod-product-compliance
Lightning Source LLC
Chambersburg PA
CBHW081320180526
45170CB00007B/2792